THE BIOLOGY OF HUMAN REPRODUCTION

by J. J. HEAD

Drawings by CYNTHIA CLARKE

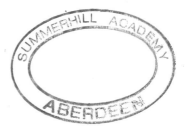

CORRIGENDA

In Figures 12, 33 and 44:
    for Humerus *read* Femur

(*Head: The Biology of Human Reproduction*)

John Murray 50 Albemarle Street London

ISBN (John Murray) 0 7195 3706 1
ISBN (USA and Canada) 0 9503903 1 3

Filmset and printed in Great Britain by
BAS Printers Limited, Over Wallop, Hampshire, England.

Acknowledgements

The author is grateful to John Murray (Publishers) Ltd., 50 Albemarle Street, London W1X 4BD for permission to use the following drawings from his book *How Human Life Begins*: Figs. 10, 12, 14, 17, 18, 28, 34, 37(a) and (b), 40, 41, 42, 43, 45, 46, 47, 48, 49, 51, 53, 55. Thanks are also due to the following persons and organizations: Carnegie Institute, Figs. 22, 23, 24, 25, 26, 27, 28, 54; Eagle Films, Figs. 5, 21, 32; Dr. R. G. Edwards, Figs. 6, 8; Professor D. W. Fawcett, Fig. 4; *Family Doctor*, Fig. 50; Professor A. Glauert, Fig. 3; the late Professor W. Hamilton, Figs. 29, 30, 31, 38, 39, 52, 56; A. Ironside, Fig. 44; Eurfron Gwynne Jones, Fig. 36; President of the Royal College of Surgeons of England, Fig. 33; Professor G. Rhodin, Fig. 2; Professor L. B. Shettles, Fig. 7; South Western Optical Instruments, Figs. 1, 11, 19. Cover photo of a 14 week human fetus one and one-half times life size taken by Miss M. A. Hudson and reproduced by permission of the Charing Cross Hospital Medical School, London.

Available in the United States of America and in Canada by mail order from Carolina Biological Supply Company, Burlington, North Carolina 27215; Gladstone, Oregon 97027.

There are about four thousand million human beings alive in the world today, and the number is increasing rapidly. Around 125 million babies are born each year; this works out to about two hundred and forty every minute.

A baby has first to be *conceived* by its two parents. It then develops inside its mother's body for an average time of 267 days, that is 38 weeks or nine calendar months. This time is called the *gestation period*. The baby is then born.

Cells, sex cells, and the zygote

The body is largely composed of cells. There are about one hundred different kinds of human cell. Examples that spring to mind are nerve cells, muscle cells, blood cells, bone cells, and sex cells. Fig. 1 is a photograph of a stained human blood smear, showing three different kinds of white blood cell (stained blue). These have prominent nuclei. The smaller red cells are the only cells in the body to have no nucleus when they are mature, though they have one while they are being formed in the red bone marrow. Blood cells are separate from each other, lying in liquid blood plasma. Most of the body's cells are joined to each other by connective tissue, for example the kidney cells in Fig. 2. Such cells can only be seen under a microscope by making sections of the tissue. A section may or may not pass through the nucleus. In some of the cells in this preparation it has, in others it has not.

The nucleus contains the chromosomes which in turn contain most of the genes. These are coded instructions "telling" the cytoplasm of the cell how to make proteins. It is believed that all the cells of the body except the sex cells have nuclei that are genetically identical. Despite this, various cells develop in different ways—into nerve cells or blood cells, for example. Also cells become grouped together to form tissues such as nerve tissue in the brain, muscle tissue, and bone tissue.

Tissues are often arranged into organs, like the eye, the femur (thigh bone), or the stomach. Nearly all the information "telling" the developing organism how to do these things is contained in the *genetic code,* the DNA, of the nuclei of cells.

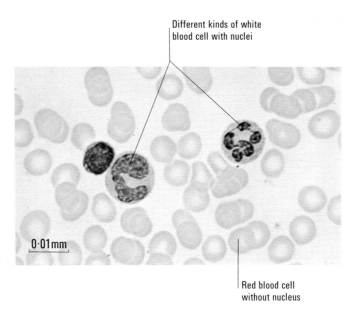

Different kinds of white blood cell with nuclei

0·01mm

Red blood cell without nucleus

Figure 1. Human blood cells

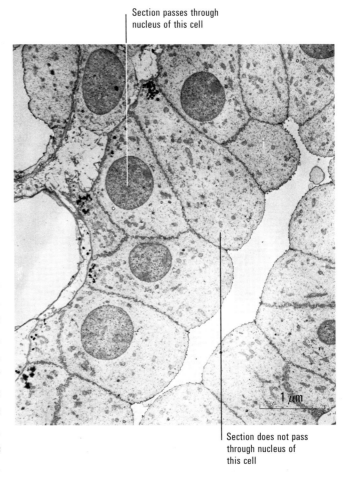

Section passes through nucleus of this cell

1 μm

Section does not pass through nucleus of this cell

Figure 2. Section of human kidney cells

1

A human being starts life as a single cell with a single nucleus containing 46 chromosomes. It is called the *zygote*, from a Greek word meaning "joined." This is because it is formed by the joining or fusing of two sex cells, the *sperm*, made by the father, and the *ovum*, made by the mother. The nuclei of sperm and of ovum contain only 23 chromosomes each, so the zygote contains 46, like all the other body cells.

Sperm

Like blood cells, sperms are suspended in liquid and are not joined to each other. The mixture of sperms and liquid is called *semen*. One cubic centimeter of human semen contains about 20 million sperms.

Sperms are little more than a swimming nucleus. Fig. 3 shows some guinea pig sperms (sperms of all mammals have the same basic structure). The dark staining nucleus is capped by an *acrosome*, which shows up brightly in this photograph. The acrosome contains digestive enzymes which enable a sperm to dissolve a small hole in the wall of the ovum and so enter it. Below the nucleus is the *midpiece*, and beyond that the *tail*. The total length of a human sperm from tip to tail is about three hundredths of a millimeter. Fig. 4 is a longitudinal section of part of a bat sperm. It shows much more detail than Fig. 3. Note the acrosome and the nucleus. The upper part of the mid-piece is a single mitochondrion coiled round and round. The sperm contains no food reserves. The mitochondrion provides chemical energy (ATP) for the sperm to move. It makes ATP by oxidizing sugars obtained from the liquid part of the semen. Human sperms can live and swim for about twenty-four hours after a man has deposited semen inside a woman's body.

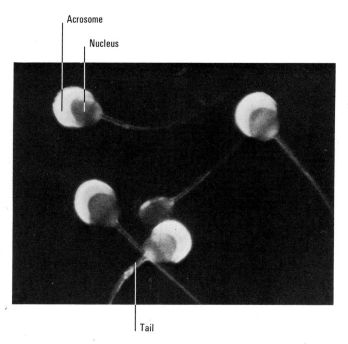

Figure 3. Guinea pig sperms

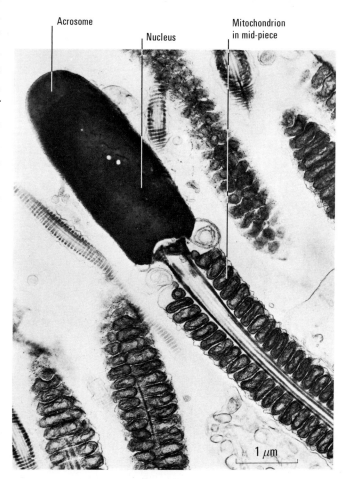

Figure 4. Longitudinal section of part of a bat sperm.

2

Ovum

A human ovum is shaped like a ball and is about one-tenth of a millimeter in diameter. It does not swim. As well as its nucleus it contains food reserves which help to nourish the embryo in its earliest stages of development. There is a marked difference in the number of sperms made by boys and men, and of ova (plural of ovum) made by girls and women. In his early teens a boy reaches a stage of development when his testes start to make sperms. This is called *puberty*. He goes on making billions of sperms for the rest of his life. By contrast, a newborn baby girl already contains all the ova she will ever make. There are about half a million ova in each of her ovaries. At the age of puberty, her two ovaries start to shed one egg per calendar month. Around age 49 they cease to do this. This time is called the *menopause* or *change of life*. Thus she sheds a total of about 800 ova in her life; the rest of her one million ova degenerate.

Fig. 5 shows part of a human ovum surrounded by sperms. Fig. 6 shows three human sperms lying outside the wall of an ovum, one about to penetrate by dissolving a hole in its wall. Fig. 7 shows a human sperm moving inside a human ovum.

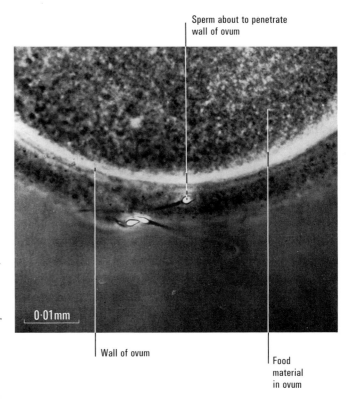

Figure 6. Part of a human ovum, sperm about to penetrate the wall.

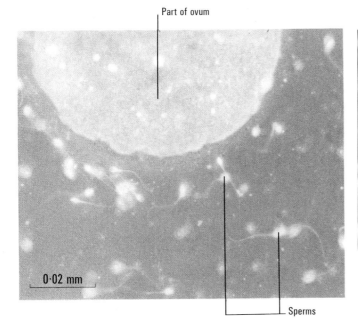

Figure 5. Part of a human ovum surrounded by sperms

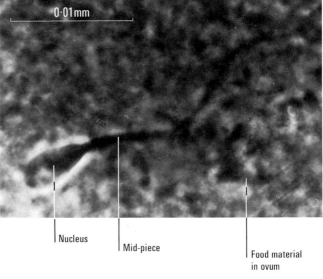

Figure 7. Human sperm moving inside a human ovum.

Zygote

In Fig. 8 we see a human ovum containing two nuclei. One is the ovum nucleus. The other looks very much like it, and not like the head of a sperm. It has, however, been formed from a sperm nucleus which has swollen and is about to fuse with the ovum nucleus. This nuclear fusion is called *fertilization* or *conception*. The cell is no longer an ovum, because its nucleus now contains 23 + 23 = 46 chromosomes, whereas the ovum nucleus contained 23. The fertilized ovum is called the zygote, and from it about 200 million cells develop before the baby is born.

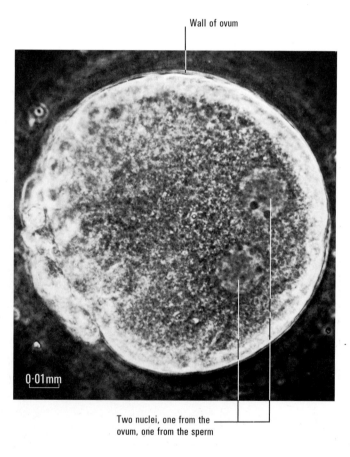

Wall of ovum

0·01mm

Two nuclei, one from the ovum, one from the sperm

Figure 8. Human ovum just before fusion of sperm and ovum nuclei.

Where the sex cells are made

The man

Sperms are made in the man's two *testes* (Fig. 9). These are oval and hang outside his body in a sac of skin called the *scrotum*. This skin is unusual in that it contains large numbers of muscle fibers. When the man's body is warm, these muscle fibers relax. The testes then hang away from his body, as shown in Fig. 9. In other conditions—cold, or fear, or when a man is about to ejaculate semen into a woman—the muscle fibers contract and draw the testes close to his body.

Fig. 10 shows one testis removed from the scrotum. Inside it is divided into some 250 compartments. Each contains between one and four long twisted tubes, within which the sperms are made. If all the tubes were unraveled and laid end to end they would measure about 250 meters. The small tubes lead into a mass of larger tubes collectively called the *epididymis*. This lies beside the testis (Fig. 18) and acts as a store for sperms made in the testis tubes. The sperms do not swim to the epididymis but are moved there from the testis tubes. Leading from the epididymis is a single tube, the sperm duct or *vas deferens*. This goes upward into the man's body. We will trace its path later.

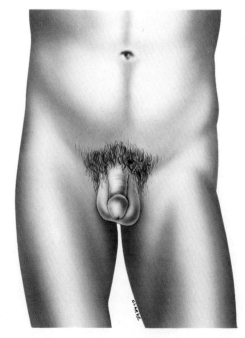

Figure 9. Drawing of human penis, scrotum, testes, and pubic hair.

4

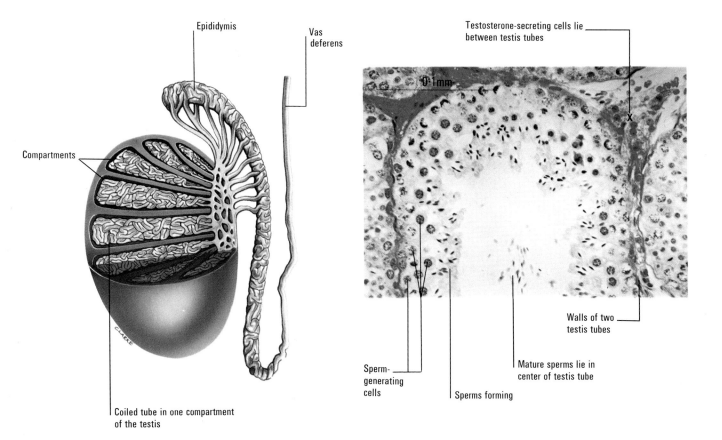

Figure 10. Human testis dissected to show internal structure. Epididymis and vas deferens also shown.

Figure 11. Transverse section of part of a human testis tube.

Fig. 11 shows a transverse section of one testis tube. The cells at the edge are dividing and making sperms, some of which can be seen lying free in the liquid-filled center of the tube.

Aside from its primary function of making sperms, the testis plays an important part in sexual development. Lying between the sperm-producing tubes, in the region marked X in Fig. 11, are hormone-secreting cells. When a boy reaches puberty these cells secrete a hormone *testosterone* which has many important effects on the development of his body. It causes him to become more muscular, to develop more body hair, including pubic hair and facial hair. It also causes growth of his larynx (voice box), and so breaking of the voice; and it causes his penis to grow bigger.

The woman

The woman's sexual organs are all inside her body. Fig. 12 shows their position. They consist of the two ovaries (which make the ova), the two *Fallopian tubes*, the womb (*uterus*), and the birth canal (*vagina*).

These organs are located low down in the woman's hip basin. Her ovaries are at the back of her body. In Fig. 12 all the other internal organs have been omitted for clarity.

As with the testis of a man, the ovary of a woman has two functions, one of making the sex cells (ova), the other of making hormones. The hormones are called *estrogens* and *progesterone*. Estrogens are responsible for causing fat to be deposited under her skin, and this helps to produce the characteristic shape of a woman and to conceal muscles which are more readily visible through the skin of a man.

Estrogens also cause growth of her breasts and growth of body hair under her armpits and in the pubic region. They also cause the lining of her womb to grow. This is important because of menstruation, the discharge of blood from the womb each month (p.13). Progesterone is primarily responsible for maintaining pregnancy by preparing the lining of the womb (the *endometrium*) for the reception of a developing zygote.

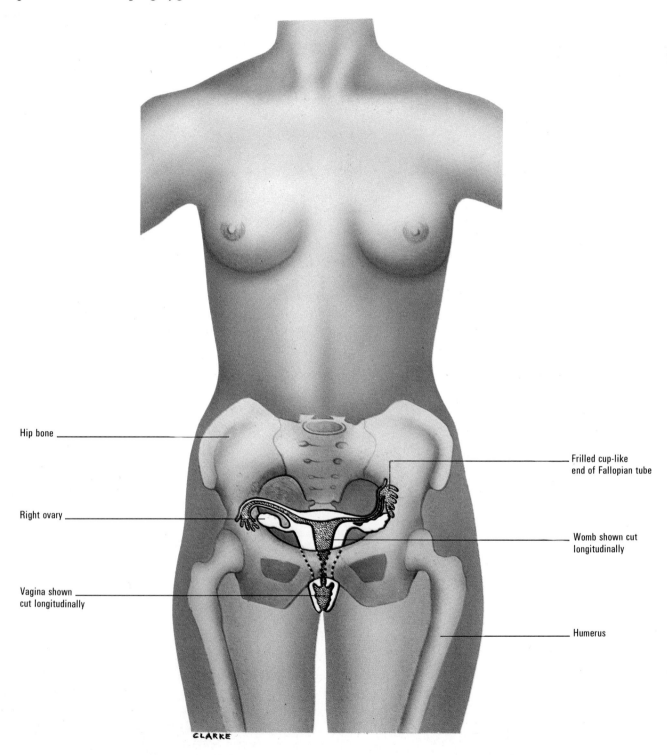

Figure 12. The position of the sexual organs in a woman's body.

Fig. 13 is a drawing of a section through a woman's ovary. When a girl reaches the age of puberty at about 13 years, a monthly cycle of events takes place in her ovaries. Several ova out of the half million present in each ovary at birth associate with each other and become surrounded by a group of cells. The group forms a cavity within itself and is called a *Graafian follicle*. The cells lining the follicle secrete estrogens. After about fourteen days the ovum is dischared through the surface of the ovary. This is called *ovulation*. The follicle now collapses. Over the next few days it develops into a *yellow body* which secretes estrogens and progesterone. Together these prepare the lining of the womb to receive a developing zygote. An ovum is capable of being fertilized for up to 36 hours after ovulation, so the woman can only become pregnant if the man has deposited semen in her body at this particular time.

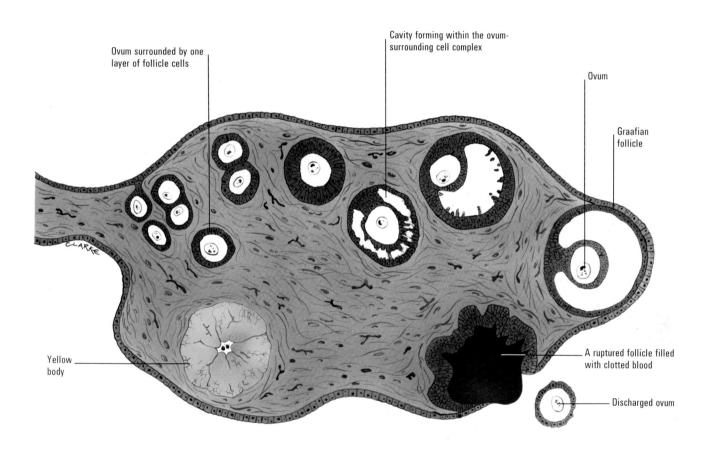

Figure 13. Growth of Graafian follicle, ovulation, and formation of yellow body.

Fig. 14 shows some of these events as a diagram. The left ovary is drawn as it appears from the outside. The right ovary is drawn in section, like Fig. 13. When the ovum is discharged (ovulation), the frilled cup-like end of the Fallopian tube moves and clasps the ovary so the ovum passes directly into it. Toward the base of the drawing we see the top of the vagina leading to the neck (*cervix*) of the womb. Several sperms have been drawn here, much enlarged.

A man discharges, or *ejaculates* 60 to 100 million sperms each time he has sexual intercourse. It is thought that only a few thousand of these gain access to the womb and swim up the Fallopian tube. Details of human fertilization are unknown, for they cannot be observed in a living person. Only one sperm is needed to penetrate the ovum and produce fertilization. Once this has happened, any other sperms around the ovum cease attempting to penetrate. However, it seems that a large number of sperms must surround the ovum in order for the one to penetrate, and if a man produces less than about 35 million sperms in the semen he ejaculates, he is likely to be infertile.

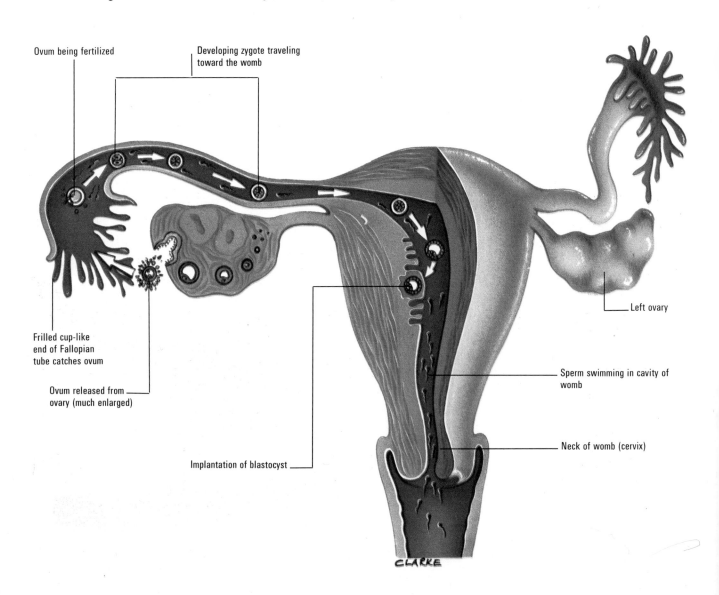

Figure 14. The vagina, womb, ovaries and Fallopian tubes, shown intact on woman's left side, in section on her right side. Ovulation, fertilization, and implantation are illustrated on her right side.

8

Fig. 14 shows fertilization. The cavity of the Fallopian tube is filled with liquid, and the cells lining it are covered with minute hairs which move together and produce tiny currents which carry the zygote onward toward the womb. This journey takes between four and seven days. Meanwhile the lining (endometrium) of the womb thickens and secretes liquid ready to receive the developing embryo. Estrogen and progesterone cause this to happen. While being moved toward the womb, the single-celled zygote starts to divide and by the time it arrives it has formed a hollow ball consisting of about 130 cells.

Copulation

When a man and a woman create a child they nearly always have feelings of love and tenderness for each other. Usually they share their whole lives in marriage.

Making a baby together is a large part of their love for each other as well as for the new child. It brings them into a special physical closeness, for the man's erect penis is inserted into the woman's vagina. This is called copulation, or making love, or sexual intercourse.

To understand how the parents' sexual organs are involved in copulation, we must first look more closely at them.

A woman's sexual organs are all inside her body. From the outside, only her pubic hair can be seen (Fig. 15). Her vagina (birth canal) opens to the exterior at the slit-shaped *vulva*, but this is concealed by pubic hair in Fig. 15. Fig. 16 is a drawing showing the sides of the vulva, the entrance to the vagina, parted. To obtain this viewpoint the artist has imagined the woman lying down with her legs parted—they would extend outward from the page. We can see that the vulva is bordered by two sets of lips, the *labia majora* on the outside and the *labia minora* within them. At the apex of the labia minora is the woman's clitoris.

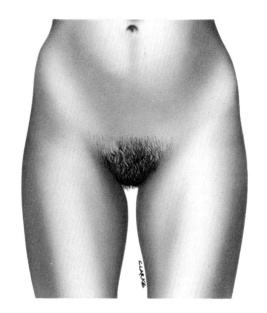

Figure 15. Drawing of the pubic region of a woman.

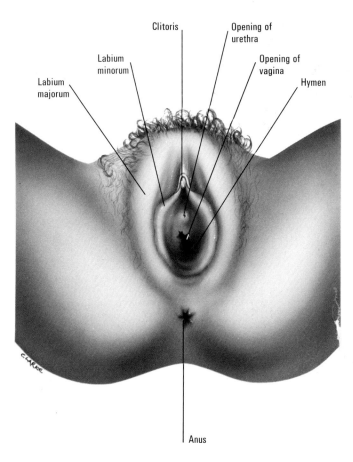

Figure 16. Pubic region of a woman, with the labia parted.

9

Before a woman has ever had sexual intercourse the entrance to her vagina is partly or sometimes completely closed by a thin fold of skin called the *hymen*. This varies a lot in shape, and may be absent altogether. It is pushed aside by the man's penis during her first sexual intercourse and does not grow back over again.

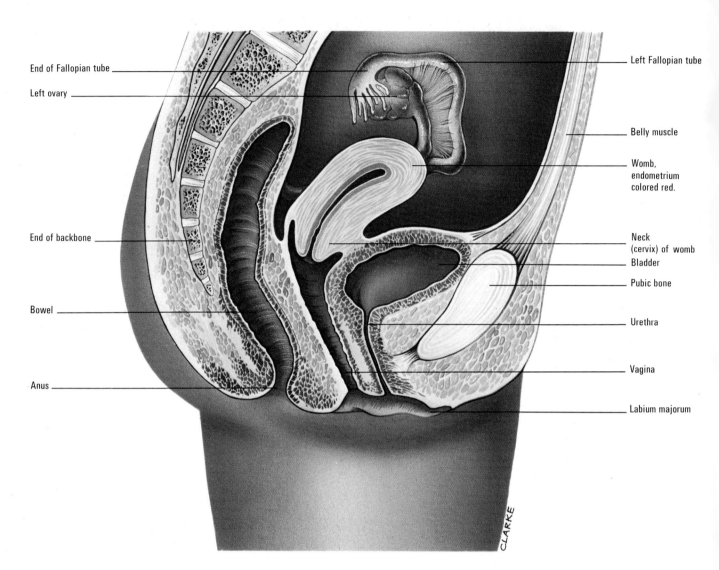

End of Fallopian tube

Left ovary

End of backbone

Bowel

Anus

Left Fallopian tube

Belly muscle

Womb, endometrium colored red.

Neck (cervix) of womb

Bladder

Pubic bone

Urethra

Vagina

Labium majorum

CLARKE

Figure 17. Section through center part of a woman's body, showing sexual and other organs.

Fig. 17 helps us to understand how the sexual organs lie inside the woman's body, and their relationships to some of her other organs. Note first the frilled end of her Fallopian tube clasping her ovary. Next her womb, with its lining, the endometrium, shown in red. The neck (cervix) of her womb is at the top of her vagina. At the bottom of her vagina we can see her left labium majorum.

The other organs in her abdomen have been left out of the drawing, notably her large and small intestines. We should note, however, that her bladder lies in front of her womb and vagina, and that it has a separate duct, her *urethra*, leading to the outside. Find the opening of the urethra in Fig. 16. Behind her vagina and in front of her backbone is her bowel, ending at her anus.

Thus when the baby has developed in its mother's womb and is being born, it must pass between her backbone and her pubic bone to reach the outside world.

Fig. 18 shows us the middle part of a man's body cut in half lengthways. We have already seen the testes, the scrotum, and the penis, and can now follow how these link up with his internal sexual organs.

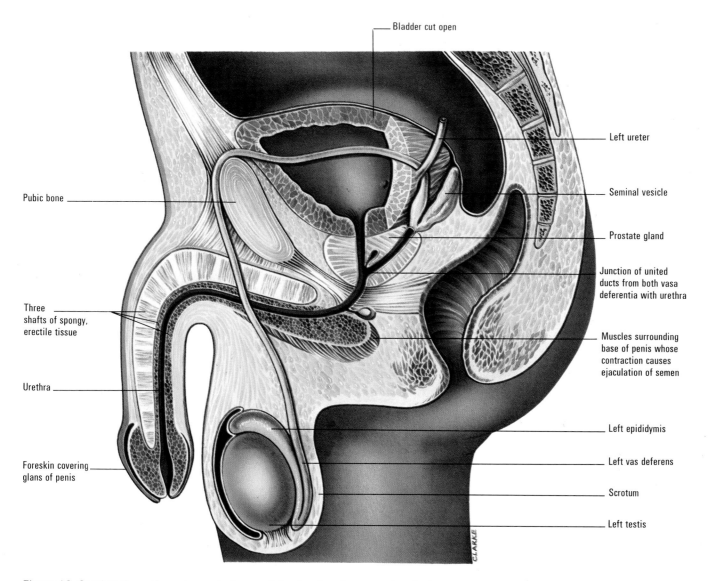

Figure 18. Section through center part of a man's body, showing sexual and other organs.

First find his testis. The one drawn is his left testis. At the back of it lies his left epididymis, and leading off from this his left sperm duct or vas deferens. Trace this up into his body. It passes over the front of his pubic bone and curls round his left *ureter*. The ureter is the tube bringing urine from the kidney to the bladder. Since the bladder has been drawn cut away, we can see the small hole on the other side where his right ureter enters his bladder. Leading out from the bottom of the bladder is his urethra. This has been colored brown and is easy to follow along the length of his penis to the exterior.

Just below his bladder a tube leads into his urethra. This has been formed by the joining of the vas deferens from each side. There are also two important glands, the seminal vesicle (one to each side toward the end of each vas deferens), and the prostate gland. The latter is a single gland surrounding the upper part of the urethra and the ducts leading into it from each vas deferens. Find these glands in Fig. 18.

The figure also shows that the penis consists largely of spongy tissue surrounded by skin. At the apex, or *glans* of the penis, the skin is free, forming the foreskin. This is often cut off by the doctor shortly after birth in a small operation called *circumcision*.

Fig. 19 is a transverse section of the penis of a man. It contains three shafts of spongy tissue, and the urethra is surrounded by the one that lies nearest the man's body when his penis is soft, as it is in Figs. 9 and 18. These three shafts are shown more clearly in the drawing of a dissection of the penis in Fig. 20 The spongy tissue contains many blood spaces. When blood is delivered to the penis faster than it can be drained away, the penis enlarges and becomes *erect*. As well as increasing in length and girth, it becomes hard and no longer hangs down but points up so that the urethra is now facing away from the man's body. It cannot be bent downward when in this condition because the spongy tissue extends backward under the pubic bone (Fig. 18). Neither can urine be passed through it.

The penis can now be inserted into the woman's vagina. Moving his penis in the vagina causes the man to ejaculate, that is to shoot semen out of his penis with considerable force. First the sperms stored in each epididymis are moved up each vas deferens. They do not swim, and are immobile at this stage. They are squeezed along by muscular contractions of the wall of the vas deferens (a similar peristaltic contraction to that which moves food along the intestines). The sperms collect at the point where the two vasa deferentia join the urethra, surrounded by the prostate gland. This place is marked in Fig. 18. Secretions are added from the two seminal vesicles and from the prostate gland. These contain sugars and other chemicals, and the sperms start to swim in the liquid, which is now semen. The duct in which the semen is collecting becomes distended.

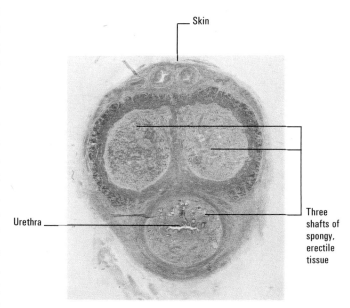

Figure 19. Transverse section through a man's penis.

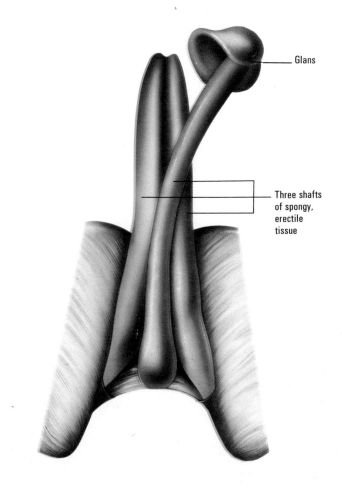

Figure 20. Dissection of human penis to show the erectile shafts.

12

At the base of the penis lies a group of strong muscles. They are colored purple in Fig. 18. The man reaches a stage when this group of muscles contracts very strongly eight or ten times. This causes 3 to 5 cm³ of semen to be flung out of the top of his penis. This is called *orgasm*. He can control its onset voluntarily, but once it has started he cannot control it. His semen is deposited at the neck (cervix) of the womb. Some of the sperms gain entrance and start to swim into the cavity of the womb and into the Fallopian tubes. If the woman has ovulated at the right time, some of the sperms may encounter an ovum, and fertilization may take place (Fig. 14).

Menstruation

Before following the development of the zygote, we must pause to mention an important aspect of a woman's life, menstruation, or monthly period.

We noted on p. 7 that when an ovum is shed from the ovary, the Graafian follicle becomes converted into the yellow body and this secretes estrogens and progesterone (Fig. 13). If the ovum is fertilized, the yellow body continues to secrete, keeping the lining of the womb, the endometrium, in a state to receive the developing embryo and to retain it once it has become attached to the endometrium. Fertilization may, however, not take place. Obviously it will not if the woman has not had sexual intercourse with a man; and even if she has fertilization may not have occured. In that event, the yellow body degenerates and ceases to secrete estrogen and progesterone. The endometrium now dies and is cast off. This is called menstruation.

The endometrium is 2–3mm thick and contains many blood capillaries. An adult woman loses between 50 and 500 cm³ of blood at each menstruation, which may last for four to five days. The age when menstruation starts is very variable, though in the United States at the present time the average age is fourteen. Menstruation ceases after the menopause.

Development of the zygote

As soon as the nuclei of the two sex cells have united to form a zygote (Fig. 8), this single cell starts to divide. Each of the daughter cells divides, giving four cells. Each of these divides, giving eight cells. These three stages are shown for a monkey zygote in Fig. 21.

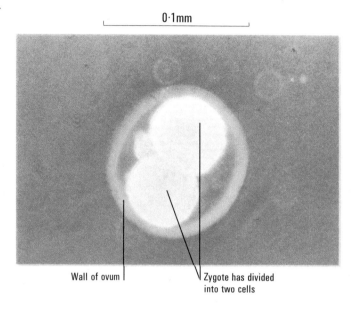

0·1mm

Wall of ovum   Zygote has divided into two cells

Figure 21 (a). Monkey zygote after first cell division.

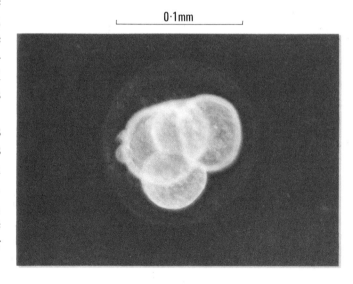

0·1mm

Figure 21 (b). Monkey zygote after second cell division.

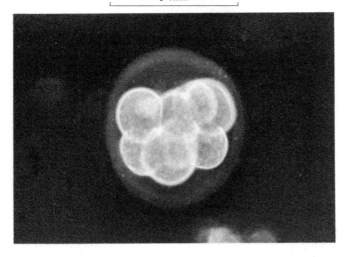

Figure 21 (c). Monkey zygote after third cell division—eight cells present inside wall of ovum.

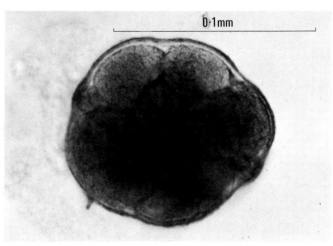

Figure 23. Developing human zygote with about 18 cells inside the wall of the ovum.

Fig. 22 shows a human zygote that has divided giving two cells. The nucleus of each shows clearly. So also does the wall of the ovum. Cell division has not increased the size of the developing zygote. Fig. 23 shows a developing human zygote with about 18 cells in it, all contained within the wall of the original ovum. By the time the developing zygote reaches the wall of the womb it consists of about 130 cells arranged like a hollow ball and called a *blastocyst*. Fig. 24. is a section cut through this ball.

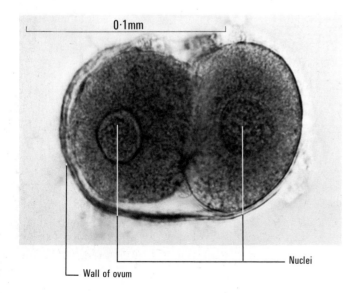

Figure 22. Human zygote after the first division.

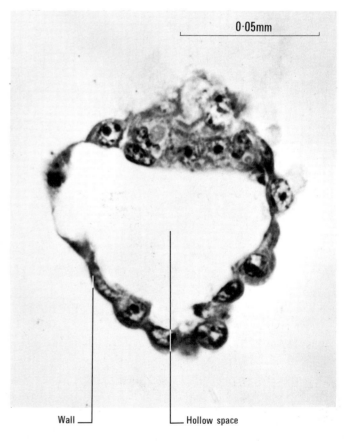

Figure 24. Section through a human blastocyst.

The outside of the ball is sticky, and attaches to the endometrium. Fig. 25 is an outside view of a human blastocyst adhering to the endometrium.

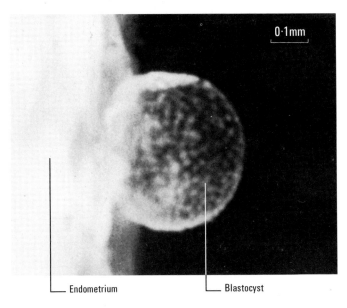

Figure 25. Human blastocyst attached to the endometrium.

Fig. 26 is a longitudinal section of a similar blastocyst. It is attached to the endometrium at one point and already shows differentiation into an *inner cell mass,* which will give rise to the baby and the umbilical cord, and a *wall.* The wall will develop into the *chorion,* a shaggy outer coat surrounding the space in which the baby is developing. The part of the chorion next to the wall of the womb develops into the *placenta* (Fig. 40).

The blastocyst is less than half a millimeter in diameter. It sheds the wall of the ovum, which still surrounds it. Now it sinks into the soft endometrium, a process called *implantation.* Sinking is probably due in part to digestive enzymes secreted by the blastocyst. These dissolve cells of the endometrium. However, the endometrium grows over the blastocyst as well. Fig. 27 is a surface view of a blastocyst which has just become implanted and is covered by a thin layer of endometrial cells.

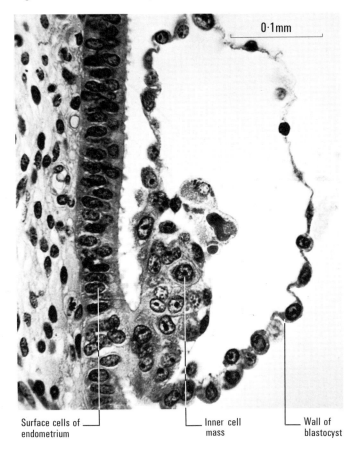

Figure 26. Longitudinal section through human blastocyst attached to endometrium.

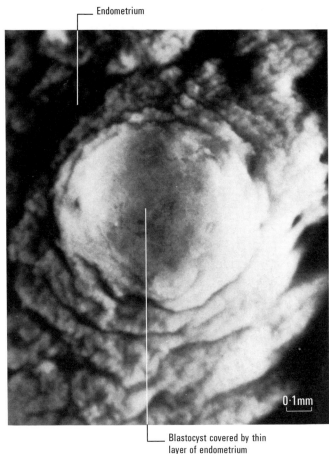

Figure 27. Implanted human blastocyst covered by thin layer of endometrium, seen from above.

15

Figure 28 is a vertical section through an implanted blastocyst. When a blastocyst has become implanted the woman is said to be *pregnant*, or *with child*, or *carrying a baby*.

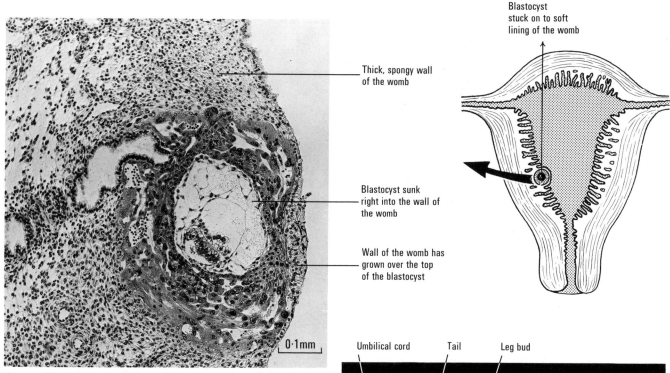

Thick, spongy wall of the womb

Blastocyst sunk right into the wall of the womb

Wall of the womb has grown over the top of the blastocyst

Blastocyst stuck on to soft lining of the womb

Figure 28. Vertical section through an implanted human blastocyst.

Changes in form as the baby develops

It is the inner cell mass (Fig. 26) that develops into the baby and its umbilical cord. Its dividing cells rapidly assume different forms, becoming nerve cells, muscle cells, blood cells, and so on. These form tissues such as brain tissue and muscle tissue, and tissues differentiate into organs like the eye, the heart, the brain, the bones, and many others. Outwardly the developing baby changes its form rapidly. Fig. 29 shows a developing baby five weeks after fertilization of the ovum, that is about one month after implantation. It is recognisably human, though it has a tail. Fig. 30 shows a developing baby three weeks later, eight weeks after fertilization of the ovum. There has been much further development. Its head now shows the eyes and ears clearly, and the arm and leg "buds" have the beginnings of fingers and toes.

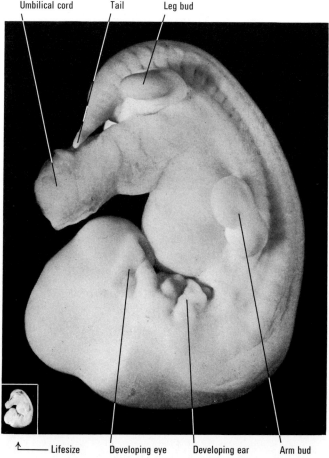

Umbilical cord   Tail   Leg bud

Lifesize   Developing eye   Developing ear   Arm bud

Figure 29. Developing baby five weeks after fertilization.

16

Most of the baby's internal organs have started their development by this stage. It already has its own developing heart, arteries, veins and lungs.

Umbilical cord   Leg bud   Arm bud

Developing eye   Developing ear

Figure 30. Developing human baby eight weeks after fertilization.

absorber, protecting the baby from any jolts to its mother's abdomen. The liquid also helps to keep the baby at an even temperature.

The outer membrane is the chorion. The part of it next to the womb develops into the placenta. In Fig. 31 it is lying behind the developing baby, and has masses of shaggy blood vessels. The part of the chorion on the observer's side was removed before this photograph was taken. The amnion surrounding a 16 week old developing baby is shown in Fig. 32—here again the chorion has been removed.

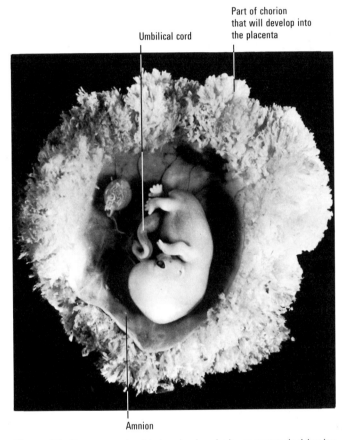

Umbilical cord   Part of chorion that will develop into the placenta

Amnion

Figure 31. Seven week old developing baby surrounded by its amnion. Part of its chorion is shown behind it.

Chorion and amnion

Meantime the wall of the blastocyst has developed into two membranes or "skins" which surround the developing baby. Fig. 37(b) shows them diagrammatically. The inner one is called the *amnion*. Fig. 31 shows it surrounding a seven week old developing baby. The amnion is filled with fluid, the *amniotic fluid* or "waters". These act as a shock

17

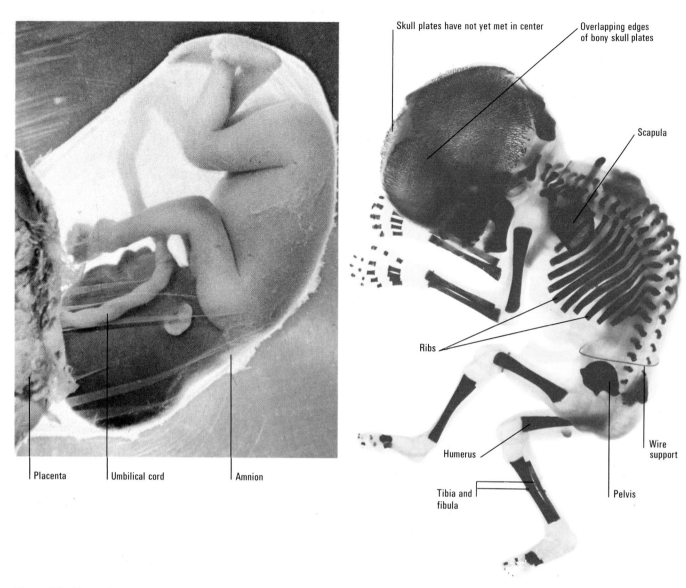

Figure 32. 16 week old developing baby in its amnion.

Figure 33. Stained skeleton of 14 week old developing baby.

The baby's skeleton

Fig. 33 shows the skeleton of a baby fourteen weeks after fertilization of the ovum. The baby had died, and its bones were stained with red dye. It already has its backbone, ribs, pelvis, and shoulder blades. Note that its tail has disappeared. Also visible are its arms and legs, its palms and fingers, and the corresponding foot bones. Wrist and ankle bones have not yet appeared. Its skull consists of developing bony plates which overlap each other and do not meet at the top. This is still

so at *term,* the time when the baby is born, and its head is capable of changing shape somewhat when being pushed through its mother's birth canal.

Compare Fig. 33 with Fig. 34, a drawing of an adult skeleton. Are there any other bones that have not yet developed in the 14 week baby's skeleton?

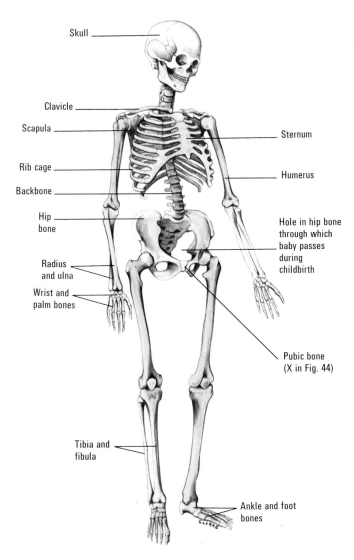

Skull

Clavicle

Scapula

Rib cage

Backbone

Hip bone

Radius and ulna

Wrist and palm bones

Sternum

Humerus

Hole in hip bone through which baby passes during childbirth

Pubic bone (X in Fig. 44)

Tibia and fibula

Ankle and foot bones

Figure 34. Drawing of an adult skeleton.

is seven months old it can usually be kept alive in an incubator (Fig. 36). Here it is warm and is fed on drops of milk. If it is not seven months old at birth it usually dies.

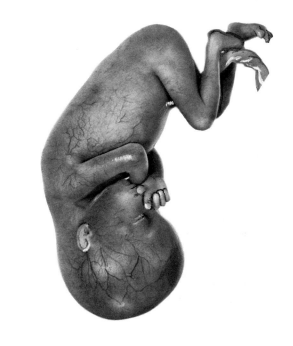

Figure 35. Developing baby five months after fertilization (half natural size)

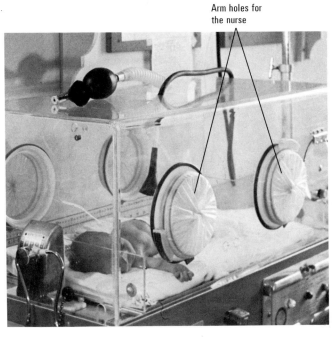

Arm holes for the nurse

Figure 36. Premature baby in an incubator.

Miscarriage

The baby is born nine calendar months (forty weeks) after fertilization. At the beginning of the sixth month (Fig. 35), it is very like a newborn baby except that it is very thin. The mother can now feel the baby moving inside her, and it has times when it is awake and times when it sleeps. Its heartbeat can be heard through the wall of its mother's abdomen. Occasionally the placenta may become unstuck and the baby may be born *prematurely*. This is called *miscarriage*. If the baby

19

A seven month developing baby weighs about one kilogram, and during the last two months in its mother's womb it puts on about two and one-half more kilograms, mostly fat which keeps it warm after birth. The outside world is much colder than the inside of the mother's womb.

It is sometimes hard to remember how very small a developing baby is in its early stages. The two drawings in Fig. 37 are life size. Fig. 37(a) shows the developing baby three weeks after fertilization, and Fig. 37(b) five weeks after fertilization. Note how the amnion and chorion project into the cavity of the womb, nearly filling it. Fig. 38 shows an actual eight-week baby in position in the womb, life size.

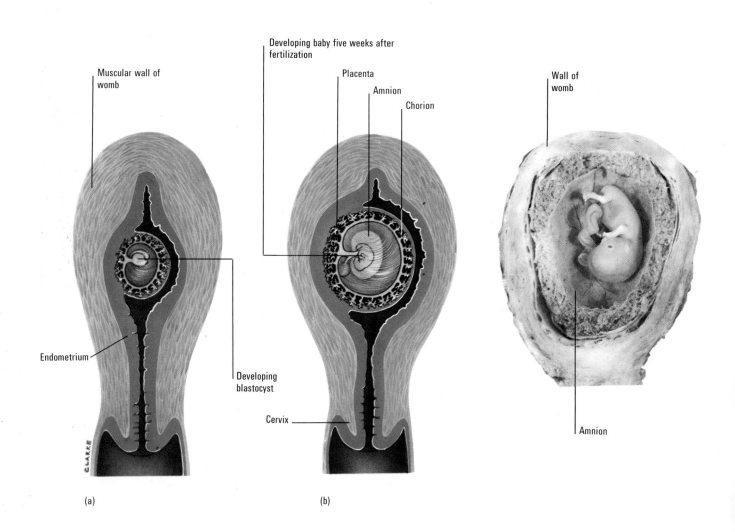

(a)   (b)

Figure 37(a) and (b). The womb and developing baby (a) three (b) five weeks after fertilization, drawn life-size.

Figure 38 (far right). Eight-week baby in the womb, life-size.

20

Feeding the developing baby

When a human baby is born its body contains some two hundred million cells. It started life as one cell, the zygote, which weighed a fraction of a gram. The newborn baby weighs about three and a half kilograms. For this increase to take place the developing baby must be supplied with food. It also needs oxygen to obtain energy by the oxidation of sugars and fats, but it neither feeds nor breathes. The alveoli of its lungs are in any case crumpled and do not expand until the first breath is taken. While in the womb the baby makes no breathing movements with its chest or diaphragm.

The baby also needs to excrete the waste chemicals it makes, notably carbon dioxide and urea. All these functions, feeding, oxygen supply, and the removal of wastes, are carried out on behalf of the developing baby by its mother. She feeds for it, breathes for it, and excretes for it. These processes take place by means of the placenta. Fig. 39 is a photograph of a full-grown placenta. It is about the size of a dinner plate. Note the umbilical cord, which shows that this view of the placenta must be of the surface facing the baby and not the surface facing the wall of the womb. Comparison with Fig. 40 will make this point clear.

The developing baby is joined to the placenta by the umbilical cord, which consists of three large blood vessels surrounded by a jelly (Fig. 52). Two of the blood vessels are called the *umbilical arteries*. At the end of the second month of its development, the baby has its own circulation, and this is much like that of the adult except first little blood is sent to its lungs, which do not function, and second, all its blood is carried along its umbilical arteries to the placenta. This blood has given up its oxygen and dissolved food substances to the baby. It is therefore deoxygenated. As it is traveling away from the baby's heart, the vessel containing it must be called an artery, but since the blood is deoxygenated, this artery should be colored blue in diagrams. This is the reverse of the normal way of showing arteries in red.

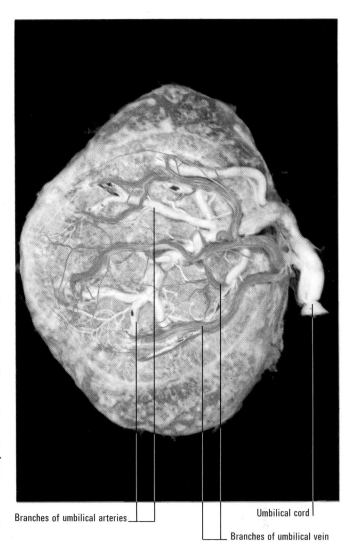

Branches of umbilical arteries

Umbilical cord

Branches of umbilical vein

Figure 39. A mature placenta. Note the umbilical cord, which must have faced the baby. Branches of umbilical arteries injected with yellow dye, branches of umbilical vein injected with red dye.

21

Fig. 40 shows a two-month-old baby in position with the wall of the womb and the placenta cut across. Fig. 41 is a close-up view of part of Fig. 40. Note the blood arriving from the baby in the two umbilical arteries, and shown in blue. These arteries branch and form tufts of capillaries which lie in large blood spaces in the placenta. The mother's blood is delivered to these spaces by arteries branching directly from her aorta and therefore containing much oxygen in the form of oxyhemoglobin in her red blood cells. It is drained away from the spaces into her veins.

Thus in the blood spaces the baby's blood is separated from its mother's blood only by the thin wall of the capillary tuft in which it is traveling. Dissolved foods and oxygen diffuse from the mother's blood across the capillaries into the baby's blood. The baby's waste substances, mostly carbon dioxide and urea, diffuse outward from the capillaries into the mother's blood and are taken into her circulation to be excreted by her lungs and her kidneys. The baby's blood, replenished with dissolved foods and oxygen, travels back to its body in the umbilical vein. This vessel is called a vein because the blood in it is moving toward the baby's heart, but since it is oxygenated blood we must reverse the normal way of coloring it and show it as red (Fig. 41).

These processes of exchange between mother and baby are very rapid and substantial. The volume of the mature placenta is about 500 cm³ of which about 350 cm³ are occupied by the capillary tufts on the baby's side. The total length of the tufts is about 50 kilometers, and their total surface area—the surface through which exchange is taking place—is about 14 square meters. The area of skin on an average adult man is 2 square meters, and a comparison of these figures shows the extensiveness of the area provided for food, oxygen, and waste exchange between the mother and the developing baby. About 500 cm³ of the mother's blood passes through her placenta each minute under resting conditions, approximately one tenth of the output of her heart. All the baby's blood (400 cm³) passes through the placenta each minute.

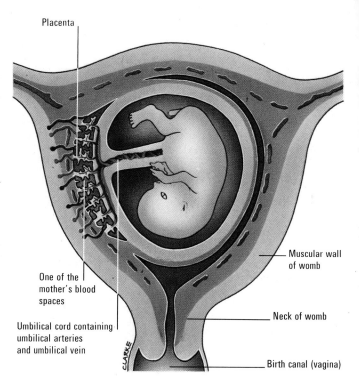

Figure 40. Section through the womb, showing the placenta to which the two month old developing baby is attached by its umbilical cord.

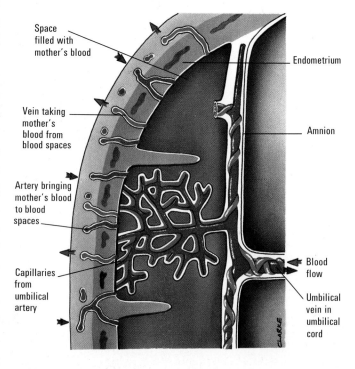

Figure 41. Detail of Fig. 40 showing the maternal blood spaces in the placenta, the capillary tufts, and the umbilical cord.

22

Changes in the mother's abdomen during pregnancy

While the developing baby grows, so does its mother's womb. At the start of pregnancy the womb weighs about fifty grams and is about seven centimeters long. At the end of pregnancy its weight, not counting its contents of the baby, amnion, chorion, amniotic fluid, and placenta, is about two kilograms, an increase of some forty times. It is now approximately thirty five centimeters long. After the baby is born it returns to its former small size.

These changes are shown in Figs. 42 and 43. Fig. 42(a) shows the outline of the womb at the following times after implantation: 0·3 months, 4,5,6,7,8, and 9 months. Fig. 42(b) shows the outline of the mature womb, with the Fallopian tubes and ovaries. Fig. 42(c) shows outlines of the womb as it decreases in size after the first, third, fifth, seventh and ninth *days* following childbirth.

Some of the increase in size is allowed for by squashing the mother's internal organs. In particular, her intestines and liver are pushed up against her diaphragm, and she may get short of breath if she exerts herself in late pregnancy, say by climbing a flight of stairs. But her belly muscles also stretch and grow, and her belly bulges outward. A side view (Fig. 43) shows the outline position of the top of the womb after three, four, five, six, seven, and eight months of pregnancy. During the ninth, last, month, the baby, the womb, and the mother's belly muscles all move downward. The complete encircled dashed line shows this stage. Look also at Figs. 45 and 46. These show the enlargement of the womb after eight months of pregnancy, and also of the mother's breasts in preparation for the milk she will produce to feed her newborn baby.

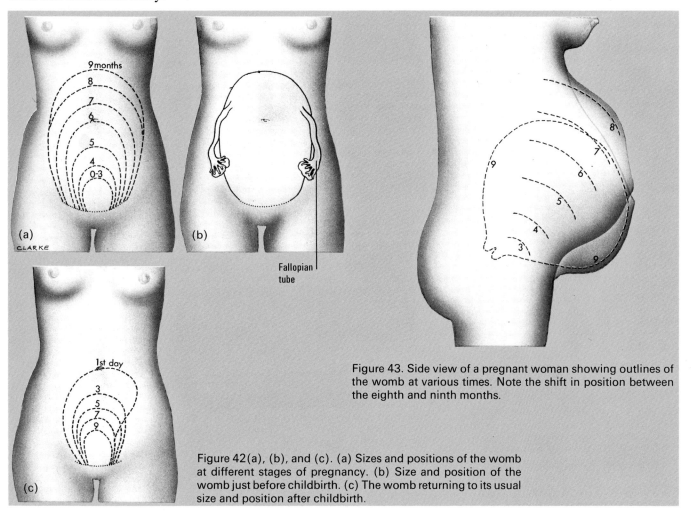

Figure 43. Side view of a pregnant woman showing outlines of the womb at various times. Note the shift in position between the eighth and ninth months.

Figure 42(a), (b), and (c). (a) Sizes and positions of the womb at different stages of pregnancy. (b) Size and position of the womb just before childbirth. (c) The womb returning to its usual size and position after childbirth.

Childbirth (labor)

The normal position of the baby in the later stages of pregnancy is upside down with its head resting in its mother's hip basin. The way out from the womb is along the vagina (birth canal). Fig. 44 is a photograph of the hip basin. It is formed from the bottom end of the backbone and the large, flared hip bones. At the front these join at the *pubic symphysis,* marked X in the figure. Three tubes pass through the hip basin (Fig. 45). From the back forwards these are the *rectum* (bowel), the vagina, and the urethra. Comparison of Figs. 44 and 46 show that to be born the baby must pass through the vagina, and although this can stretch the bones of the hip basin cannot. The largest part of the baby is its head, and this must pass through the rim of the hip basin. We noted on p.18 that the skull plates are slightly moveable at this stage, so the head, the first part to emerge, can change its shape slightly during childbirth.

A woman's first childbirth takes an average time of fourteen hours, subsequent ones about eight hours. It can be painful for the mother, though this can be relieved if the mother relaxes. Many women are taught how to do this at prenatal classes. Some women use a mild anesthetic ("gas and air").

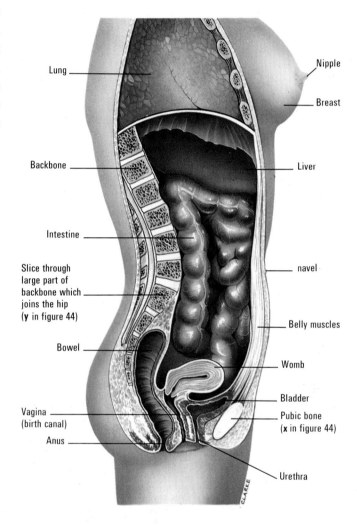

Figure 44. Skeleton of the hip and upper leg. Arrow shows path traversed by baby between backbone and pubic symphysis during childbirth.

Figure 45. Vertical section showing the position of various organs in a woman who is not pregnant. Compare with Fig 46.

24

First stage of labor

Fig. 47 shows the baby just before childbirth. Its mother is lying on her back. The baby is facing her right side and its legs are drawn up to its belly with its knees crossed, so that it takes up the least possible amount of room. Babies lie like this for months after birth, and many adults sleep in a similar position, with knees drawn up to belly. The baby is still surrounded by amnion, chorion, and amniotic fluid. One side of its head is pressed against its mother's bladder, the other against her bowel, the top against her cervix.

The womb is almost entirely made of muscle, and this contracts every few minutes throughout pregnancy. When labor starts the contractions become more frequent and stronger. They press the baby's head against the cervix, slowly stretching it open. This takes between eight and ten hours on average, and when it is complete the vagina forms a continuous open canal from top to bottom.

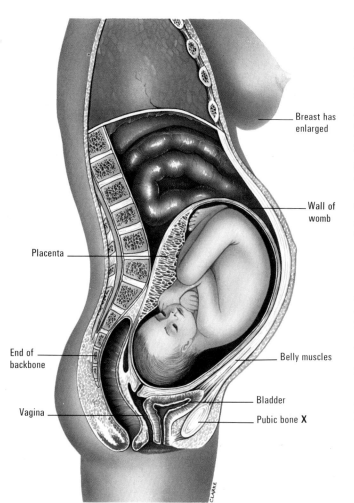

Breast has enlarged

Wall of womb

Placenta

End of backbone

Belly muscles

Vagina

Bladder

Pubic bone **X**

Figure 46. A similar view to Fig. 45, showing a woman who is eight months pregnant. Note compression of intestines and liver.

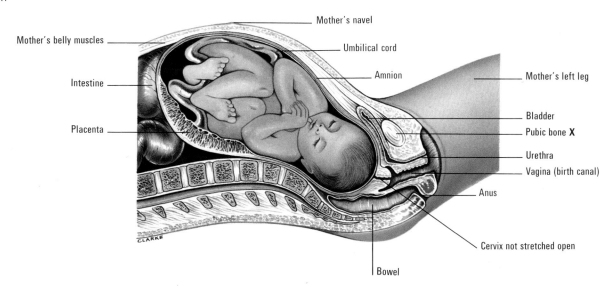

Mother's navel

Mother's belly muscles

Umbilical cord

Intestine

Amnion

Mother's left leg

Placenta

Bladder

Pubic bone **X**

Urethra

Vagina (birth canal)

Anus

Cervix not stretched open

Bowel

Figure 47. The baby in the womb just before childbirth.

25

Fig. 48 shows the cervix being stretched open. The baby's head is becoming molded to fit the birth canal.

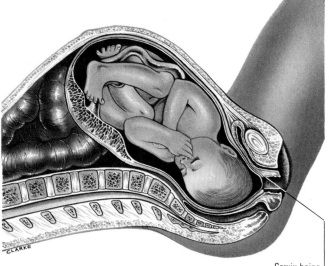

Figure 48. First stage of labor.

Cervix being stretched

Second stage of labor

This lasts from the time that the cervix is fully stretched until the baby is completely born. The emerging baby's head stretches the vagina. This stage, which lasts for about one hour, is shown in Fig. 49. Note that the baby has turned round so that it can slip more easily through the hip basin. The baby is pushed by further contractions of the womb and also by the mother pushing down with her abdominal muscles.

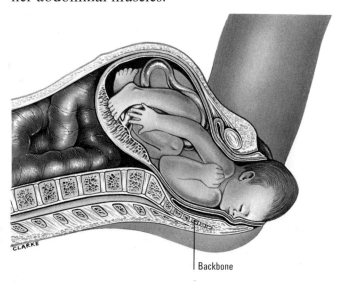

Backbone

Figure 49. Second stage of labor

At some time during the first or second stages, the chorion and amnion are ruptured, and the amniotic fluid gushes out. Once the baby's head has emerged it requires only a few more pushes to force out the rest of its body.

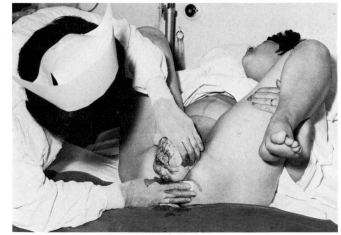

Figure 50(a). The baby's head is born.

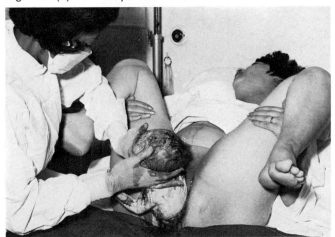

Figure 50(b). The baby's body emerges.

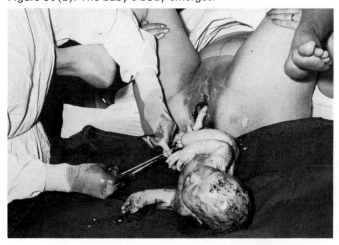

Figure 50(c). Clamping the cord. Note the mother's labia.

Third stage of labor

The baby starts to breathe with its own lungs as soon as it is born, but it is still connected to the placenta by the umbilical cord, which is long enough to allow this (Fig. 50(c)). The amnion and chorion are also still inside the womb. The cord is clamped and tied in two places and then cut between (Fig. 50(c)). The baby, now completely free from its mother, is wrapped up and removed to a cot.

About five minutes later the womb contracts again, expelling placenta, the remains of the umbilical cord, the amnion, and the chorion. These are collectively known as the *afterbirth* (Fig. 51).

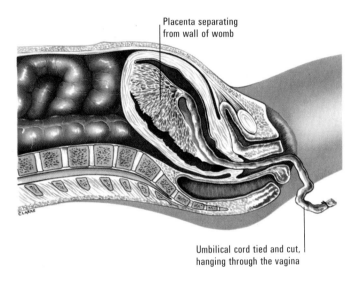

Figure 51. Separation of the afterbirth.

When the placenta separates from the wall the mother loses about 200 cm³ of blood. The open vessels in the part formerly occupied by the placenta are closed first by kinking action of the contractions of the womb, then by the normal blood clotting mechanisms. This area is, however, obviously open to infection by bacteria. Until the end of the nineteenth century, childbirth was one of the greatest hazards to human life, and many women died as a result of infection of the womb, the disease being known as *puerperal fever*. Today strict standards of cleanliness are adopted during childbirth, as can be seen in Fig. 50, and peurperal fever is almost unknown in civilized countries.

The baby is born covered in a whitish cream and a little blood. When it has been bathed, its umbilical cord is dusted and bandaged to its body. It dries up and falls away from the navel after a few days. The umbilical arteries and vein contract immediately they are cut (Fig. 52). This is very important in other mammals, whose birth is essentially the same as that of human babies. The mother bites the cord in two, and if the arteries and vein did not contract at once the young offspring would lose a lot of blood through them.

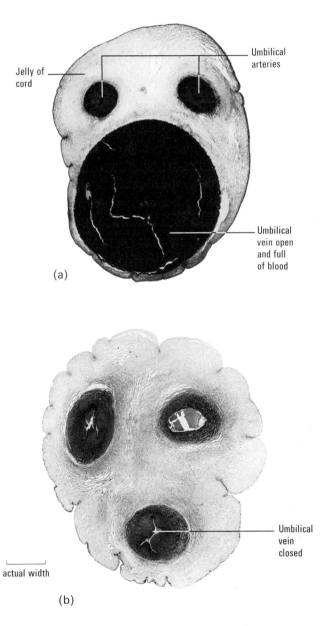

Figure 52(a) and (b). (a) Transverse section through umbilical cord before closure of umbilical vein. (b), the same after closure.

Twins

It is usual for a woman to bear only one baby at a time, but about one childbirth in 85 produces twins. One-quarter of these pairs are *identical* and three-quarters *non-identical*, and may even be of opposite sexes.

Non-identical twins arise when a woman releases two ova at the same time and both are fertilized. It is not known whether one ovary liberates two ova or each ovary liberates one. Both zygotes become implanted and develop their own amnion, chorion, and placenta (Fig. 53). Since all ova and all sperms are genetically different from each other, the two zygotes resulting from this double act of fertilization are as genetically dissimilar as if they had been conceived at different times in the mother's life and were not twins.

Identical twins arise from a single zygote. At an early stage, and for reasons that are not known, the blastocyst separates into two independent growth centers. It is impossible to observe this separation in a living person, but it probably occurs at the two cell stage (Fig. 22). Siamese twins, permanently-joined pairs of individuals, probably arise from an incomplete separation of the blastocyst at a later stage. Fig. 54 is a section through a developing human blastocyst which has already separated into two growing centers and would probably have given rise to twins. It corresponds to the stage shown in Fig. 26.

With identical twins, each baby has its own amnion, but they share the same placenta. A single chorion surrounds both amnions (Fig. 55).

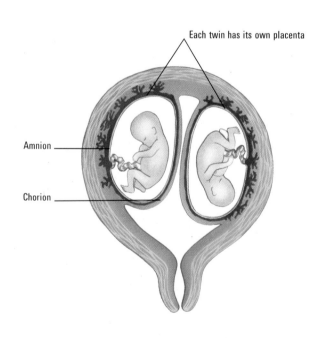

Each twin has its own placenta

Amnion

Chorion

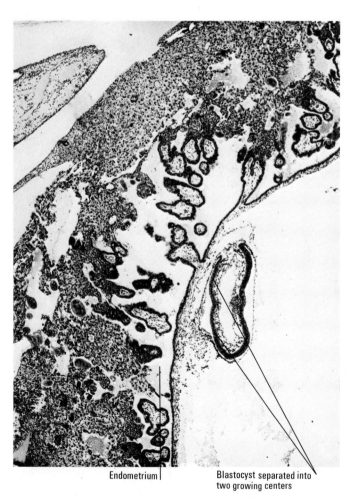

Endometrium | Blastocyst separated into two growing centers

Figure 53. Non-identical twins in the womb. Each has its own amnion, chorion, and placenta.

Figure 54. Human blastocyst that has developed two growing centers about to become implanted. Compare with Fig. 26.

28

Fig. 56 shows a pair of identical twins each with its own amnion and umbilical cord, sharing a common placenta. Identical twins are formed by the fusion of one sperm and one ovum, forming one zygote. The genetic instructions in all cells in both twins are therefore the same.

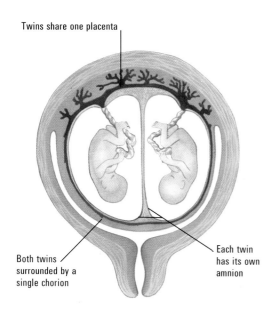

Twins share one placenta

Both twins surrounded by a single chorion

Each twin has its own amnion

Figure 55. Identical twins in the womb. Each has its own amnion, but they share one placenta and are surrounded by one chorion.

Figure 56 (below). Identical twins sharing one placenta, each surrounded by its amnion.

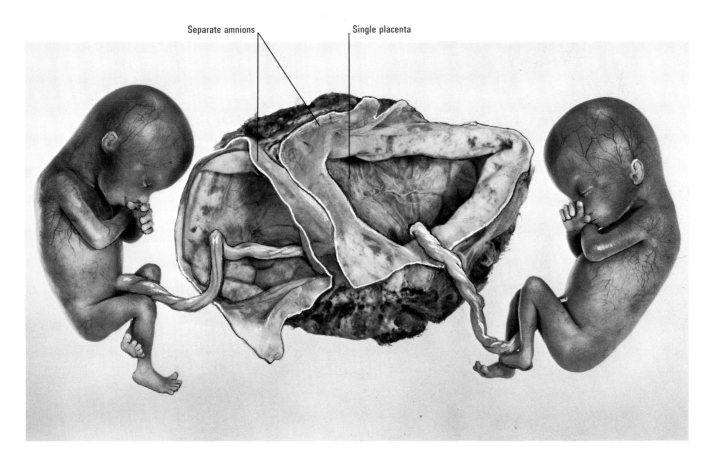

Separate amnions

Single placenta